# STRENGTH

## THE ULTIMATE GUIDE TO FAT LOSS

### Kevin Dea

# Contents

# Introduction

I want to thank you and congratulate you for purchasing the book, *"Strength - The Ultimate Guide to Fat Loss"*.

In this book, we will discuss some of the best and the most important factors that are part of fitness and fat loss training. These factors will give you the best possible results, while creating a body that is functional and can still move and get your daily tasks accomplished.

Basically, this book is for anyone that has tried everything in their search for the "perfect" body. This book is mostly targeting women, but truthfully is for anyone who just wants to look and feel better, and for anyone who just wants to get in shape and stay in shape- and even challenge themselves physically. You will learn more than you ever thought possible about fat loss and becoming the slim, trim beast you want to be!

I have personally been in the strength, conditioning, and fat loss industry for about eight years now. During that time, I've been able to become an expert by studying the experts on the topic, performing my own research, and through meeting with and training under some of the best coaches in the industry. Finally, I have logged hundreds- even thousands- of hours training and practicing these techniques both on myself and with others.

In the first chapter, we will be discussing fat loss in general versus weight loss. While many people use them interchangeably, they are actually two completely different, but similar concepts. In the next two chapters, we will be discussing the two mistakes that women commonly make when it comes to trimming down their bodies: nutrition and working out.

Then, we will discuss how our approach is different than the rest. Most programs tell you to weigh yourself on a regular basis. We do not. We tell you to look at yourself in the mirror- take before and after shots- but don't depend on the scale to track your progress.

Next, in order to be successful with this program- or any other for that matter- you must have the right mindset and goals. You must have an ultimate long term goal that you wish to achieve. However, since a long term goal can be a bit overwhelming, you must break that down into smaller, easier to achieve goals. In order to achieve your goals, you have to do something and have a "can-do" attitude. After all, no one ever did anything by sitting around doing nothing, right?

There are some things you should know about getting in shape. There are some myths and facts about getting toned and certain things you should and should not do. Also, did you know that your sleep habits could be having an effect on your fat loss journey?

Finally, we will explain more about getting started with our program and how to cultivate the winner's mindset. As I already said, you must have a winner's mindset if you expect to achieve. You must go into it already envisioning your success.

After you read this book, you will be walking away with a much better understanding of what you need to be doing in your own exercise routine. You'll have an idea of what you need to look for in a fitness program and you will know what your strongest muscle is (hint: your mind). You will be able to work through the fluff that is in some programs and boil them down to what is really important in helping you to achieve the body that you've always desired- and feel the best you ever have!

Thanks again for downloading this book, I hope you enjoy it!

# General Fat Loss

Many times, people go into the gym saying, "I want to lose x pounds by x time." It can be 10 or 15 or even 50 to 100. However, that kinds of mindset truly bothers me because you really don't want to be losing pounds just for the sake of losing pounds. Instead, you want to focus more on fat loss than simply losing pounds. In layman's terms, fat loss is getting rid of body tissue that is unwanted and is not necessary for basic human functioning, while at the same time maintaining a lean body mass- that is, your organs, muscles, bones, etc. Basically, fat loss is getting rid of the extra weight that was never meant to be there in the first place.

The truth is that everyone needs a little bit of fat, or meat on their bones. Also, women actually need more than men- believe it or not. However, you don't need as much extra as some people seem to have. Fat loss will specifically target the weight that we don't want. Honestly, fat loss can help you to gain weight in terms of the number on the scale/pounds- but still lose the fat that you wanted to get rid of.

## The Difference Between Fat Loss & Weight Loss

These days, weight loss is one of the hottest topics. It seems like everyone is trying to lose weight. However, as mentioned above, there is a difference between weight loss and fat loss, even though many people typically use the terms interchangeably. This chapter will explain the major difference between fat loss and weight loss as well as the one you need to be aiming for and how you can achieve your goals.

So, what's the difference between the two? We'll start by giving you a definition of fat loss and one for weight loss so that you can get a better perspective.

*Weight Loss*: when you want to lose weight, you want to lower your overall body weight- that is the sum of your body fat, muscles, bones, and organs.

*Fat Loss*: when you want to lose fat, you want to lower the **amount of body fat that your body is carrying.**

As you saw earlier in this chapter, women do need more body fat than men, so a good, healthy goal for body fat is 10 percent for men and around 15 percent for women.

Basically, what it boils down to is this: weight loss is simply the number you see on the scale (which is unreliable and irrelevant as you will see below) and fat loss is the way your clothes are fitting you.

So, if you find that your clothes are fitting you better after you've been working on your program, and the scale is going down at the same time- you're definitely headed down the right track with your fat loss. On the other hand, if you find that the number on the scale is decreasing but the way your clothes fit has not really changed, this isn't really very good. Chances are that you're losing tissue that your body needs instead of the fat that it really does not need.

## Weight Loss Problems

If you're trying to lose weight, it's usually because you feel like you're carrying too much fat. There are those that have to lose weight, such as athletes when training and conditioning their bodies for a competition. However, again- they want fat loss, not weight loss.

Therefore, when you're trying to slim down and lose fat, you really should stop weighing yourself- the scale is completely unreliable. The truth is that your body weight is going to fluctuate on a daily basis. After all, since weight is the sum of your ENTIRE body- not just your fat- the number on the scale is influenced by contents of your bladder/bowels/stomach, whether you are carrying or have just lost some water weight (bloating), muscle gain and loss, and fat gain and loss. So, as you see, when you simply go by the number on your scale, you have no clue what in the world is going on.

In addition to being unreliable, the number on the scale is completely irrelevant. After all, you can have two people that are approximately the same height and weight- but they look totally different because one of them has a lower amount of body fat than the other one.

The entire Body Mass Index, or BMI, standard is flawed because it does not take your body fat into account when it's measured. Two people can have the exact same BMI, and one can be healthier than the other one because he has a lower amount of body fat.

## How Can the Scale Mislead You?

When you're trying to get started on a healthier lifestyle and lose fat, clothes, pictures, and mirrors do not lie. Fat calipers do not lie either. On the other hand, the scale can actually become one of your worst enemies. It will mislead you and completely kill your motivation. You will get discouraged and most likely just give up and remain in your unhealthy state.

Here is how the scale can be misleading and kill your motivation, causing you to give up:

1.  Carbohydrates and water: water and carbs bind together- so, yes cutting carbs from your diet can help you to lose weight. Guess what? It's simply water weight. This is why low carb diets make you lose so much weight in the first two weeks or so. On the other hand, when you increase your carbohydrate consumption, you will gain weight. Guess what? Again, it's water weight. More carbs equals more water retention.

2.  Muscle Gains/Fat Loss: you are going to gain muscle while you are losing fat once you get into strength training. However, when you step on the scale, you'll think that you're not making any progress because the number won't move- or may even go up. Your body weight won't be going down like you want it to.

Instead of depending upon the scale to track your progress, you should track your progress using fat calipers. This will prove to you that your body fat truly is going down- even though the number may not.

# How Can You Be Sure You Lose Fat Instead of Muscle?

As we already said, when you lose weight, you are losing the sum of all of your body weight- but when you lose fat, you maintain your muscles. Keep in mind that five pounds of muscles takes up much less space than five pounds of fat. Therefore, you're going to look much slimmer but may maintain your body weight because you're building muscle.

# Keys to Lose Fat- Not Muscle

If you want to ensure that you're losing fat- not muscle- you should do the following:

1.  Make yourself stronger: strength training will help you to prevent loss of muscle and build it at the same time. It will also help to stick to your diet.

2.  Make sure you're eating healthy: instead of eating those convenience foods that are full of carbohydrates and have been processed, choose whole, unprocessed foods ninety percent of the time. Check out the eight rules of nutrition.

If you want to speed up fat loss, you can add metabolic conditioning to your routine- but if you don't include the strength training then you'll be losing muscle as well as weight and you'll end up being what is known as "skinny-fat." This is something you definitely want to avoid.

# How to Efficiently Track Progress

When you're on the path to losing fat, you don't need to be tracking your progress on a weekly basis. The changes in your weight are not going to be drastic enough. Instead, measure your progress every two weeks.

Do not weigh yourself on a daily basis. Your weight is going to fluctuate on a daily basis and those fluctuations are going to ruin your motivation. Instead, weigh yourself once every two weeks- and no more.

Stop staring at yourself in the mirror. Issues with your self-image are going to skew your perception of how you're doing. Instead, shoot full body pictures and then compare them with the old ones. If possible, consider wearing the same outfit each time so that you can see (and feel) the difference in how your clothes are going to fit- after all, the proof is in the way your clothes are fitting, not in the number on the scale.

Do keep an eye on your body fat. Purchase a fat caliper and- every two weeks- track your body fat. This will give you a much better idea of how much fat you are losing instead of stepping on the scale to see that even though you're trimming down, you're gaining weight.

Do take measurements of your body. Take the time to measure the girth of your chest, neck, waist, thighs, and arms. Your waist should be going down, but the rest should be going up.

Take pictures of yourself (or have someone do it for you). As mentioned above, these should be full body pictures from your neck to your ankles- from the front, back and side. Do this every two weeks. This will give you a better idea of how you're doing than looking in the mirror or stepping on the scale.

Keep track of your strength stats. Take the time to log your workouts. Gaining strength means that you're also gaining muscle. In addition, strength training will prevent you from losing muscle.

Finally, pay attention to what people are saying. They are going to notice the changes in your body much more than you will. You will notice that your clothes are fitting you better- so pay attention to that as well.

Think about this- the truth may be that you may not really want to lose weight after all. Many times, big guys find that once their body fat is lowered, they don't mind being big- as long as they are healthy overall.

So, when you make the decision that you must lose weight, focus on losing fat first and foremost. Then, once you have your body fat down a bit, decide if you like what you're seeing. After that, you can decide if you still must lose weight or if you like what is looking back at you.

After all, losing fat goes together with building up muscle. When you build muscle, you're going to gain a little bit of weight- but it's muscle weight, not fat. Muscle is lean, sexy, and bent. Muscle looks amazing. You want to do whatever you can to put that on. You want to build muscle and burn fat.

So, if you just work on weight loss- simply burning and getting rid of nearly everything in your body, it's so much harder to get it off and keep it off. However, if you build muscle, you will be able to keep the fat off. Muscle allows you to burn fat much more quickly than if you were simply trying to reduce the number you see on the scale.

In the next two chapters, we will talk about some of the mistakes that people often make when it comes to losing fat. They mess up regarding nutrition and their workout.

# Where People Go Wrong with Nutrition

Too often, when it comes to weight loss/fat loss, women tend to make a few mistakes. They focus more on weight loss (that is, the number on the scale) instead of fat loss (that is their measurements).

There are two most common areas that women go wrong when it comes to losing weight/getting in shape. They are as follows:

1. Nutrition

2. Workout

The first one we are going to talk about is nutrition. As far as that goes, it's basically their preconceived notion of what they should be doing. When we go on a diet, we typically count calories. However, in my opinion, this is the wrong way to do it.

Let's look at it like this: if you are obese and you are overeating everything in sight- then yes, you need to be counting calories. On the other hand, if you are a 5'5" woman who is somewhere between 175 to 200 pounds, then you really don't need to be focused so much on counting your calories.

The problem in the second case is not so much the amount of food that is being eaten but the quality of that food. In general, women don't really understand the fact that they can eat 1,500 to 2,000 GOOD calories, such as lean proteins and green veggies and still lose fat, therefore losing the weight that they want to- WITHOUT starving themselves.

The truth is this: in order to lose fat- you really don't need to starve yourself. The only ones that must be watching what they eat are those that are overeating. Instead, we need to focus more on learning how to truly nourish our bodies and help them to recover the right way.

Recover, you ask?

Yes, when you are working out, your body needs fuel to replace what was lost in the gym. You need to rebuild and recover your bodily systems. Think about calories being to your body what gas is to a car. It keeps you going. A calorie simply informs you of miles per gallon. It's really not telling you anything about what you are actually getting out if it.

See, when you overfill your car with gas, it spills over. When we overfill our bodies with calories, it spills over onto our stomach, hips, thighs, and more- we gain fat. However, again- keep in mind that most people are not overeating at all. On the contrary, they are not eating enough.

Think about it like this: what if you never filled up your car with gas- only putting in a gallon or two at a time and your car held on to the gas for dear life because it was never sure when the next time it would be filled up. Well, that is what your body is doing. When you are not eating properly, your body grabs hold of everything you put in it, storing the fat as energy to use later on because it doesn't know when the next time you plan to eat is.

## Four-Week Eating Plan

When it comes to losing fat instead of just pounds, you must have an effective combination of protein and high fiber, this four week plan will help you to do the following:

1. Lose fat

2. Boost metabolism

3. Help build muscle

With this four week plan, you will not experience annoying hunger or crazy cravings that typically come along with simply cutting back on calories. If you wish to indulge in the holiday meals, that's perfectly fine! You can simply get yourself back on track and strip away those pounds you gain with this simple meal plan. Additionally, if you're trying hard to stay on the bandwagon, stick to this meal plan to avoid any unwanted weight gain.

# Grocery List to Get You Started

Here is a grocery list to help you to get started on this four week meal plan.

___ 1) Fresh Fruit (such as grapefruit, bananas, apples, etc)
___ 2) Eggs
___ 3) Frozen/Fresh Berries
___ 4) Whole Milk or 2% Milk
___ 5) Plain Greek Yogurt
___ 6) Large Chicken Breasts
___ 7) Organic Peanut Butter
___ 8) Old Fashioned or Steel Cut Oatmeal
___ 9) Skirt Steak
___ 10) Ground Lean Turkey Meat
___ 11) Brown Rice
___ 12) Fresh/Frozen Fish such as tilapia, salmon, etc.
___ 13) Fresh/Frozen Veggies
___ 14) Lean Deli Meat such as roast beef, turkey, etc.
___ 15) Butternut Squash
___ 16) Canned Tuna/Salmon
___ 17) Avocado
___ 18) Canned Beans such as pinto, black, lentils, and more
___ 19) Low-Fat Cheese (shredded or sliced)
___ 20) Baked/Sweet Potato

# Meal Plan for Fat Loss

Following is a week-long meal plan for fat loss. If you do this for 4 weeks, you will kickstart your metabolism and your body will begin to burn- instead of holding on to- fat. You will see that you are losing inches. If you are combining this with a great workout routine- you will most likely NOT lose overall weight because you will be gaining muscle. However, you will notice that your clothes fit better- and those fat calipers we mentioned earlier will be reading much smaller numbers.

## Breakfast Meals for Fat Loss

**Day One:**
**Spinach Shake**

**What you will need:**
- 1 cup unsweetened almond milk
- ½ banana
- 1 tablespoon organic peanut butter
- 2 scoops chocolate or vanilla whey protein powder
- 2 handfuls baby spinach
- Ice (to desired thickness)

What you will do:
Place all ingredients into a blender and blend until smooth. Pour into your favorite glass and enjoy.

**Day Two:**
**Onion, Spinach, & Feta Cheese Scramble on English Muffin**

**What you will need:**
- 2 whole eggs
- 2 egg whites
- ¼ cup each spinach (fresh or frozen) and Vidalia onion (chopped)
- 2 tablespoons feta cheese, low fat
- Salt/pepper as desired
- Bowl of steel cut or old-fashioned oatmeal

What you will do:
Scramble your eggs, adding salt/pepper as desired in a bowl. Warm medium skillet on stove and then pour eggs into it. Add spinach, onion, and feta cheese. Cook to desired consistency. While eggs are cooking, place English muffin into toaster to lightly brown. Once toaster pops up, place English muffin on plate and then egg scramble onto the English muffin. Enjoy!

**Day Three: Repeat Day One**

**Day Four:**
**Oatmeal with Strawberries**

**What you will need:**
- 1 scoop strawberry (or other flavor) protein powder
- ¾ cup cooked oats
- ½ cup banana
- 1 cup strawberries, sliced

What you will do:
Mix together banana, protein powder, and oats in a bowl. Top with strawberries. This is an excellent way to start the day!

**Day Five:**
**Yummy Berry Parfait**

**What you will need:**
- ½ cup each blueberries, blackberries, and cherries
- ½ cup plain Greek yogurt, low fat
- ¼ cup vanilla Greek yogurt, low fat
- ¾ cup steel cut or old fashioned oats

What you will do:
Get out your favorite parfait glass. Mix together both kinds of yogurt. This will give it a light, not overpowering, vanilla flavor. Layer fruit, yogurt, and cereal. Enjoy!

Day Six:
Blueberry Oatmeal Pancakes
** Keep in mind, this recipe serves six people.

What you will need:
- 6 beaten egg whites
- 2 teaspoon oil
- 1 teaspoon each vanilla extract, baking powder, and cinnamon
- 1 cup milk, skim
- 2 ½ cups oats, old-fashioned
- 1 cup blueberries
- ½ cup applesauce, unsweetened
- Nonstick cooking spray

What you will do:
Place all ingredients, except blueberries, into a blender and mix until you reach typical consistency of pancake mix. Then, very gently fold blueberries in. Heat your skillet to medium heat and coat with cooking spray. Pour ½ cup batter on skillet to make each pancake. Then, cook flipping each one once to ensure that both sides are a golden brown color.

Day Seven:
Yummy Breakfast Omelet

What you will need:
- 2 whole eggs
- 2 egg whites
- 1 small jalapeno, seeded and minced
- 1 teaspoon hot sauce
- 2 teaspoon red onion, chopped
- ¼ cup black beans (be sure to rinse)
- Salt/pepper to taste
- 2 tablespoon low-fat Mexican cheese blend, shredded
- Nonstick cooking spray

What you will do:
In a bowl, combine the hot sauce, onion, and jalapeno. Spray skillet with cooking spray and heat on medium heat. Cook your eggs, seasoning with salt/pepper as desired. Stir in your cheese and black beans.. Top with hot sauce, onion, and jalapeno mixture. Then, roll into a burrito. If desired, serve with salsa on side.

# Lunch Meals for Fat Loss

During the day, you're usually busy and on-the-go, so you want something that is quick and easy. Too often, this translates into running through the drive thru somewhere and getting something that's not at all healthy. The key to fat loss is sticking to an eating plan that promotes your metabolism and overall health. Following are 7 days of lunch meals that will do just that.

Day One:
- Chicken Salad with Tropical Twist
- What you will need:
- 2 tablespoons chopped water chestnuts
- 1 cooked and shredded chicken breast, large
- 1/3 cup each mango and pineapple
- ¼ cup cottage cheese, low fat
- 1 ounce almonds
- 2 cups spinach
- Few avocado slices

What you will do:
Mix together all ingredients except avocado and crackers. Then, serve with avocado. Enjoy!

Day Two:
- Tuna Salad and Minestrone Soup
- What you will need:
- 1 cup minestrone soup
- 2 tablespoon mayonnaise
- 1 teaspoon whole grain mustard

2 can tuna (canned in water, not oil)
Sliced tomato
Sliced lettuce

What you will do:
Mix together tuna, mustard, and mayonnaise in a bowl and set aside.
Heat Minestrone soup either in microwave or on stove- whichever
you desire. Place tuna mixture onto plate and top with lettuce and
tomato. Enjoy!

Day Three:
Chicken and Roasted Veggies

What you will need:
- ½ cup tomato sauce
- 1 cup each  chopped veggies such as zucchini, mushrooms, egg-
  plant, and broccoli
- ¼ cup part-skim mozzarella cheese, shredded
- 1 large chicken breast
- 1 teaspoon red pepper flakes
- Nonstick cooking spray
- Salt/pepper as desired

What you will do:
Start by spraying your baking sheet with nonstick cooking spray.
Then, place chicken breast and veggies onto baking sheet, seasoning
with salt/pepper as desired. Spray veggies and chicken with nonstick
cooking spray. Top chicken and veggies with tomato sauce. Bake for
20 to 25 minutes at 350 degrees or until chicken is cooked through.
When there's five minutes left in the cooking process, top with cheese
and allow to melt until ready.

Day Four:
Chicken/Red Onion Quesadilla and Salad

What you will need:
- 1/3 cup balsamic vinegar

- ¼ cup cheddar cheese, low fat
- 1 large boneless skinless chicken breast, cooked/shredded
- ¼ cup thinly sliced red onion
- 2 whole wheat, high-fiber tortillas
- 1 teaspoon light dressing

What you will do:
Combine together vinegar and onions in a bowl and allow to marinate for approximately five minutes. Then, drain and set onions aside. Spray large skillet with cooking spray and heat on medium heat. Once pan is hot, add onions and cook for five to seven minutes or until onions have softened. Transfer to bowl and set aside. To warm tortillas, place in large nonstick skillet on medium heat. They will overlap and that's fine. Warm for approximately 45 seconds on each side. Sprinkle cheese on each one. Then, add chicken and sprinkle with the onions. Fold each one in half, gently pressing with spatula in order to flatten. Cook for about two minutes, or until cheese has begun to melt. Flip and cook for one to two minutes or until second side is golden brown. Serve with mixed greens and light dressing.

Day Five:
Greek Salad Bowl

- 1 teaspoon olive oil
- ½ teaspoon each oregano, garlic, and red pepper (red pepper should be diced)
- 4-6 ounces cooked, cubed steak or chicken
- 2 tablespoons feta cheese, low fat
- ¼ cup halved cherry tomatoes
- Salt/pepper to taste
- F-factor Tzatziki sauce
- **F-Factor Tzatziki Sauce
- ¼ cup Greek yogurt, plain
- ½ diced cucumber
- Dill, minced parsley, lemon juice, salt/pepper to taste

What you will do:
Combine all ingredients in a bowl. Serve with F-factor Tzatziki sauce. For Tzatziki sauce, combine all ingredients into a bowl and serve beside salad.

Day Six:
Turkey Chili and Rice Bowl

What you will need:
- ½ cup each ground/lean turkey breast, red kidney beans, drained, water
- ¼ cup each chopped green pepper, onion, and red tomato
- ¼ cup brown rice
- 1 teaspoon chili powder
- Nonstick cooking spray
- **OPTIONAL: shredded cheddar cheese, low fat

What you will do:
Cook rice as per instructions on package and set aside. Spray saucepan with nonstick cooking spray and add ground turkey and onion. Cook until turkey is brown. Add in the remaining ingredients and bring to a boil. Decrease heat to low and simmer until thick. Add rice and serve. If desired, add cheese on top.

Day Seven:
- Simple Salad
- Mixed Greens
- ¼ cup butternut squash
- 1 serving grilled chicken
- Mushrooms, cabbage, hearts of palm, tomato, beets, artichoke, asparagus, broccoli
- 1 ounce almonds
- 2 tablespoons light balsamic vinaigrette

What you will do:
Toss together ingredients in bowl with the vinaigrette. Serve with whole wheat, high-fiber crackers.

# Dinner Meals for Fat Loss

**Day One:**
**Shrimp Stir Fry**

**What you will need:**
- ½ pound shrimp, cooked
- ½ bag frozen stir fry veggies (whatever you desire)
- Salt/pepper to taste
- 2 tablespoons soy sauce, low sodium
- ½ cup brown rice, cooked

**What you will do:**
Toss all ingredients (except rice) into wok and cook. Serve over brown rice. Enjoy!

**Day Two:**
**Garlic Chicken Breast**

**What you will need:**
- 1 chicken breast, large
- 1/8 cup skim milk
- 1 teaspoon lemon juice
- 1 teaspoon tabasco sauce
- ¼ garlic clove
- ¼ cup bread crumbs, whole wheat
- ½ cup couscous, whole wheat
- 1 cup summer squash/zucchini medley

**What you will do:**
Combine all ingredients except veggie medley and couscous in plastic bag. Toss and coat chicken. Bake for about twenty minutes on 350 degree heat. Serve with couscous and veggie medley.

**Day Three:**
**Baked Crunchy Tilapia**

**What you will need:**
- 6 ounces tilapia
- 3 tablespoons high fiber bran cereal
- 1 cup sautéed high fiber veggies such as carrots, broccoli, and asparagus
- 1 small sweet potato, baked

What you will do:
Top tilapia with crushed bran cereal, as a breading. Bake until done. Serve with sweet potato and veggies.

**Day Four: Repeat Day 1**

**Day Five:**
**Salmon and Mixed Veggie Quinoa**

**What you will need:**
- 6 ounces salmon, baked
- Salt/pepper to taste
- Fresh lemon juice
- ½ cup quinoa
- 1 cup mixed veggies

What you will do:
Bake salmon to your preference, seasoning with lemon juice, salt, and pepper. Cook quinoa as per directions. Sautee mixed veggies. Serve and enjoy!

**Day Six:**
**Steak & Potatoes**

**What you will need:**
- 5 ounces skirt steak
- 1 small potato
- 1 cup broccoli
- 2 tablespoons sour cream, non-fat
- Chives

What you will do:
Cook and season steak to your preference. Bake potato. Steam broccoli. Top potato with sour cream and chives. Serve.

## Day Seven: Repeat Day 3

Substitutions for Weeks 2 through 4
After week one, chances are you'll get bored with eating the same thing all the time. However, after week one, you are allowed to make a few changes in the menu, making sure that all your meals as exciting as possible.

# Substitutions for Breakfast

Breakfast Substitution 1:
Oatmeal and Eggs the Easy Way

What you will need:
- 3 eggs
- 1 tablespoon milk
- Salt/pepper to taste
- 1 cup berries
- ½ cup oatmeal

What you will do:
Spray microwave safe bowl with cooking spray. Scramble eggs, egg whites, milk, and salt/pepper. Place in microwave for 1 minute 30 seconds. Prepare oatmeal as instructed and top with berries and serve with eggs.

Breakfast Substitute 2:
Protein/Fiber Oatmeal

What you will need:
- 1 scoop protein powder
- ½ cup 2% milk
- ¾ cup oatmeal
- 1 cup berries

What you will do:
Place cereal in bowl. Top with protein powder and berries. Add milk and enjoy!

**Breakfast Substitute Three:**
**California Omelet**

**What you will need:**
- 2 eggs
- 2 egg whites
- 1 tablespoon cheese, low fat
- Sliced avocado
- ½ grapefruit
- ¼ cup tomatoes, chopped

What you will do:
Scramble eggs, egg whites, tomatoes, and cheese. Top with slices of avocado and serve with ½ grapefruit on side.

## Substitutions for Lunch

**Lunch Substitution One:**
**Salmon Patty**

**What you will need:**
- 1 can salmon (in water, not oil)
- 2 tablespoon mayo
- 2 tablespoon each salt, pepper, and onion
- Lettuce
- Tomato
- 1/3rd cup three bean salad
- ½ cup string beans, steamed

What you will do:
Mix together salmon, mayo, salt, pepper, and onion and form a patty. Place on whole grain bun and top with lettuce and tomato. Serve with steamed green beans and three bean salad.

**Lunch Substitution Three:**
**Roast Beef and Swiss Sandwich**

What you will need:
- ½ cup each onions and green peppers, grilled
- 3 ounces lean roast beef
- 1 tablespoon creamy Italian dressing
- 1 slice Swiss cheese
- 2 slices Ezekiel Bread
- Crudités, such as raw broccoli, carrots, and celery
- 2 tablespoon ranch dressing

What you will do:
Toast bread, if desired and place roast beef, onions, peppers, Swiss cheese, and Italian dressing on one piece. Place second piece on top to make a sandwich. Serve with crudités and ranch and enjoy.

# Substitutions for Dinner

### Dinner Substitution One: Chicken Taco Salad

What you will need:
- 1 large chicken breast, cooked/shredded
- 1 cup lettuce, shredded
- 1 cup tomatoes, chopped
- ½ cup black beans
- 2 tablespoons shredded cheddar cheese
- 2 tablespoon salsa

What you will do:
Cook and shred chicken breast. Add black beans, lettuce, and tomatoes and top with cheddar cheese and salsa. Serve with a side salad and dressing.

**Dinner Substitution Two:**
**Salmon Kabobs**

**What you will need:**
- 6 ounce raw salmon
- ½ red pepper
- ½ red onion
- Salt/pepper to taste
- 1 tablespoon olive oil
- Skewers
- ½ cup quinoa
- ½ cup mixed veggies

**What you will do:**
Chop raw salmon, red onion, and red pepper into chunks. Wet skewers and arrange salmon, pepper, and onion as desired. Brush with olive oil, and dust on salt and pepper. Place on grill until salmon is cooked through and veggies are soft. Serve with quinoa and mixed veggies.

**Dinner Substitution Three:**
**Turkey Dinner**

**What you will need:**
- 6 ounces herb roasted turkey
- 1 cup each mushrooms and broccoli
- ½ cup sweet potatoes, cubed

**What you will do:**
Cook turkey until done. Cook sweet potatoes until soft and steam broccoli and mushrooms. Serve and enjoy!

When it comes to losing fat, you can't just keep eating the way you are right now- you have to make some changes. Following this eating plan will help you to kick start your metabolism and start burning more fat. In the next chapter, we will discuss the mistakes women make when it comes to working out- and the best way to lose fat for good.

# Where People Go Wrong with Working Out

As we mentioned in the previous chapter, women go wrong in two different areas when it comes to fat loss:

1. Nutrition

2. Workout

In the last chapter, we covered a 4 week meal plan that can help get you on the fast track to losing fat instead of simply losing weight. The goal should be to lose inches and get healthy. When it comes to getting healthier, you can actually end up gaining weight because you're building muscle.

When it comes to working out, most women believe that cardio is the best option because it burns the most calories. After all, they go together, right? That's not the best way to think about it. The truth is that the best way to burn fat is to build muscle and use cardio as needed.

Sure, you do need to work up a sweat to maintain your health, but believe it or not, it doesn't need to be nearly as often as you might think. Women who take part in strength training at least three to four times per week end up reaping much more benefits than those who just do cardio. This is why we go to the gym and see no results- we're not eating right and we're not working out the right way.

*7 Common Mistakes Women Make*

There are very few things more discouraging than spending time and effort in the gym and not seeing any results. The truth of the matter is, if you want a trimmer and tighter core, you are going to have to do more than simply show up. Basically, it might be yourself that is getting in the way of you losing fat. Here are seven common mistakes that almost all women make when it comes to working out.

*1.  You don't refuel with protein.*

Women who take the time to drink a protein drink after their workout routine ended up gaining fat-burning muscle mass and actually lost around 50 percent more body fat than those women who did not. You might not realize this, but the first thirty minutes after your workout are the most critical because that is when your muscles are most receptive to amino acids, which are the building blocks of protein. Try to get around 30 grams of carbohydrates and 20 grams of protein.

*2.  You start your routine with cardio.*

You should be aware that in order to lose fat, you must do more than simply burn calories while you are working out. You must increase your metabolism boosting muscles. However, most of us start our routine with cardio and then by the time we get to the weights, we have lost our steam. Instead, you should be hitting the weights as soon as you get in the gym- this is the time when you have the most energy and can lift heavier weights. This means that you'll be building muscle, which will help you to burn fat.

*3.  You're not Warming Up Properly.*

Most people get in the gym and just get started right away without preparing their muscles, joints, and energy systems for activity. Skipping the warm up can lead to injury and decrease your performance in the gym by over 40%! Its best if you take at least 10-15 minutes to get a quality warm up in. Begin with some mobility work (foam rolling, joint preparation) followed by a proper dynamic warm up that either resembles the movements you are about to perform during the main workout, or overall basic human movements. Finish the warm up with some movements that activate the central nervous system to "wake up" the body such as jumps, pogo hops, mountain climbers, and short sprints.

*4.  Your weights are not heavy enough.*

In order to build more fat-burning muscle, you'll need to be challenging your muscles by lifting heavier weights. If you've been working out on a regular basis, you should be increasing your weight by bout ten percent for a few moves each time you work out. This means that if you're doing eight workouts each time, you should choose two of them and increase the weights, leaving the other six the same. Then, the following week, choose two more, so you're doing four heavier and four at your usual weight. Do this each week until all eight exercises have been increased- then start over again. However, keep in mind that if the weight increase causes your form to be compromised, you should go back to your previous weight until you can do all reps with proper form.

5. *You frequently go full throttle on your workouts.*

If you are always working out at a very high intensity, you are probably overtraining. In addition to increasing your risk of becoming injured, it can actually stall your progress. If you don't allow your body the time it needs to recover between workout sessions, your muscles are always broken down and they're not able to repair. The breaking down and repairing process is the way you build fat-burning muscle. When you work out, your body sees the breaking down as a stressor and it can cause an increase in cortisol, which results in storing instead of burning fat.

6. *You only rely on working out to help you lose fat.*

Even when you visit the gym religiously, it's really not going to be enough to help you to lose fat. In fact, research has proven that even those who spend at least 150 minutes each week participating in physical activity are still at risk for becoming obese if they spend most of the day sitting still. However, there is good news: those who say that they spend time doing non-exercise activity, such as doing extra chores or taking extra trips to the water cooler at work, have much smaller waists than those who are not active.

7. *You're not doing your intervals the correct way.*

Interval training, that is alternating between high intensity and moderate paces has been proven to speed up metabolism for around 24 hours following your workout. In fact, researchers in Australia found that women performing a 20 minute interval training workout three times a week shed 6 pounds more in a twelve week period than those who only worked out at a moderate pace for 40 minutes three times each week. Try to get at least 15 to 25 minutes of proper interval training three to four times per week. If you're new to the interval training, or you have a lot of fat to shed, start out by stationary cycling or walking- it's much easier on your joints.

## Best Workout to Lose Fat

As we have already mentioned, the best way to lose fat is with a combination of interval and strength training. Of course, it's not a revolutionary idea, but it has been proven over and over. This method will help you to crush calories, burn fat, and avoid hitting those dreaded plateaus.

Many times, women are a bit hesitant to start lifting heavy weights. They are afraid that it will lead to a thick, bulky body. However, this couldn't be further from the truth! Building muscle will activate your metabolism, which will help you to be burning calories even when you're at rest. Therefore, the more muscle your body has, the more fat you will be able to lose. Keep in mind that muscle does weigh more than fat- so even though you may be seeing the number on the scale go up- you are still losing fat. After all, check out the mirror and see how great you look in those skinny jeans!

## Workout to Lose Fat

Here is a workout to help you get started on your path to losing fat: Kettlebell Swing-Goblet Squat-Push up ladder (these exercises are explained further down in this chapter.)

*note* client should be proficient in all movements before attempting

1 Push Up
1 Goblet Squat
10 Kettlebell Swings
2 Push Ups
2 Goblet Squats

10 Kettlebell Swings
3 Push Ups
3 Goblet Squats
10 Kettlebell Swings
4 Push Ups
4 Goblet Squats
10 Kettlebell Swings
5 Push Ups
5 Goblet Squats
10 Kettlebell Swings

Take a 2 minute break, then repeat starting at the top with 5 repetitions of the push up and goblet squat, and go down to 1.

Toning workout: (L+R = left and right sides)
Repeat 3 rounds of
Single Arm Swings X10 L+R
Reverse Lunge X10 L+R
Single Arm Clean & Jerk X10 L+R
Single Arm Row X10 L+R

Things to remember…

1. **When Squatting, deadlifting, swinging, snatching, cleaning etc., you always hinge at the hips**. What does this mean? When you hinge your hips properly, the hips take the load, not the lower back. A proper hinge ensures optimum spinal alignment and transmission of force; that is, when you hinge properly, the hips do the heavy lifting and the back is kept safe.

Here's how to hinge:
    a. Maintain a flat back (never rounded or overarched)
    b. Push your hips back as far as possible
    c. Allow your knees to bend slightly but not enough that the shin begins to transfer forward.
    d. Keep your abs braced and tight.

2. **The swing** (one-handed swing pictured left, two-handed swing pictured right)

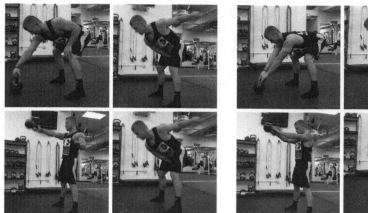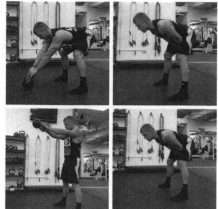

a. Stand with your feet shoulder width apart, approximately one foot behind the kettlebell you're using, and point your toes slightly outward.

b. Hinge at the hips, reach out, and grab hold of the kettlebell. Be sure to get the hips back and keep the back flat.

c. Start the swing with a forceful hike back of the kettlebell (like a football). Keep the handle above your knees at all times; this will aid in keeping your back flat. Don't hesitate with the hike. You have to throw the kettlebell back with enough force to load the hips properly for the swing.

d. When the kettlebell reaches the back of the swing, quickly and forcefully reverse the movement by squeezing your glutes, snapping your hips forward and standing up as quickly as you can. Your hips and knees should extend at the same time. Think about "jump," but without leaving the ground. The goal is to be as explosive as possible.

e. Allow the kettlebell to float between shoulder height and eye level before reversing and repeating the movement. Do not swing the kettlebell overhead. Don't lean back at the top of the swing either. Stand tall and squeeze your abs as if you were holding a plank. When done right, the kettlebell should float up at the top. The movement is powered entirely by the hips. Think about pushing a small child on a swing set. The swing is the kettlebell, your hips are the adult pushing the child (kettlebell) and your arms are the chains hanging loosely.

## 3. Goblet Squat

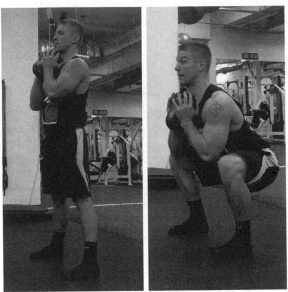

a.  Grab a kettlebell and hold it in front of your chest, like a goblet. Keep the kettlebell held close to the chest.

b.  Take a stance about shoulder width. I like to align the inside of my feet with my armpit. Screw your heels into the ground to create torque in your hips.

c.  Start the movement by hinging and then by sitting down, as if you're reaching your rear end for a bench or chair. Keep in mind that in a squat, you sit down; in a swing, you sit back.

d.  Continue to descend for as long as you're able to keep your heels on the ground, your knees in line with your toes, and your back flat. Wedge your elbows in-between your knees.

e.  When standing up, be sure that your hips and knees should extend simultaneously.

## 4. The push up:

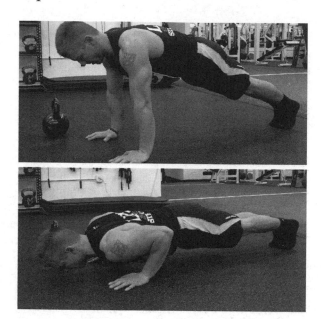

a.  Set up in the top of a push up position so your hands are directly under your shoulders and your feet are together. Screw your hands into the ground as to create torque within your shoulders.

b.  Brace your abs, acting as though they are a shield and squeeze your butt.

c.  As you lower into the push up, keep your elbows pointed back and tucked in to your sides.

d.  When you hit rock bottom push hard into the ground and drive back up into a full lockout position (elbows fully extended).

## 5. The Reverse lunge

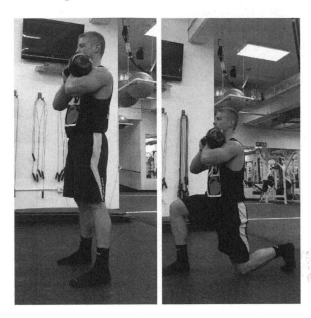

a. Take the same stance as you would for a goblet squat, with a kettlebell either in the racked position, or in the goblet position.

b. Begin by taking a large step back and maintaining the width of your stance. Keep your torso upright and rigid, don't lean forward, twist, or rotate. Avoid letting your stance narrow as well.

c. Continue to lunge until you gently touch your knee to the ground. Think about letting your knee just "kiss" the ground.

d. When you stand back up, push on both legs with equal force and return to your starting position.

## 6. The bent over row:

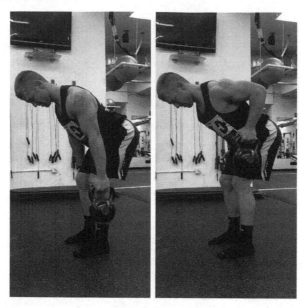

a. Set up exactly as you would for a clean or swing.

b. Grab the bell with one arm, squeezing the abs and keeping your shoulders pulled back and square with the ground.

c. Pull the bell up to your chest, keep your arm as close to the body as possible.

d. Pause at the top, with the shoulders pulled back, and then slowly press the bell back towards the ground.

## 7. The Clean & Jerk

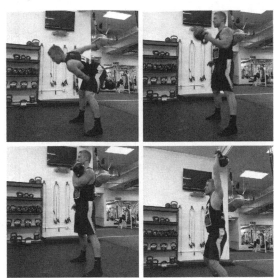

a. Position your body as if you were preparing to do a single arm swing.

b. Hike the kettlebell back between your legs like a football.

c. Snap your hips forward once it reaches the back of the hike, just as you would during a swing.

d. As the kettlebell swings forward, tuck your elbow in to your body, as if there was a strap keeping you from pulling your elbow away from the body, and redirect the bell up the center of your body. Think of the motion you perform when you zip up a winter jacket.

e. Catch the weight in the racked position.

f. Begin to take a quick dip with your hips.

g. Explode out of the dip. Think "jump" without leaving the ground.

h. As you explode, push the kettlebell up with your shoulder. While the kettlebell moves upward, quickly drop your hips down and back in to a quarter squat position. The kettlebell should be locked out overhead while in the quarter squat position.

i. Stand up with the bell locked out over head. Slowly lower the bell to the racked position and repeat.

# How is This Approach Different?

So far you've learned a lot, right? You've learned some general information about fat loss versus weight loss and why they are two totally different, but similar concepts which are sometimes confused. Then, you learned the common mistakes that women make related both to nutrition and to their workout. There are a few things you can do with both to ensure that you lose fat and build muscle.

The more muscle you build, the more effective your body will be at naturally burning fat. When you go on crazy diets- you end up making your body go into starvation mode, which is never a good thing. When your body is in starvation mode, your body holds on to fat for energy later on.

1.  This approach is different for a few different reasons:

2.  This program is based upon natural, basic human movements. We do not isolate specific muscles.

The focus of nutrition in this program is not based on calories because creating a caloric deficit is not the best way to lose fat. Sure- you'll lose weight from all over your body- but you still may be fat.

Let's take a look at the first reason that this program is different. This program does not isolate specific muscles but is based upon basic human movements. See, when we were all born, there were specific movements that were innately programmed into us. We didn't have to be taught how to do them- we basically just figured them out on our own.

However, as we grow, we lose track of those innate movements from sitting at a desk all day long at work or at school. We end up with poor posture from simply slouching on the couch at home- or anywhere else for that matter.

The truth is that poor posture is at the very basis of our problems. It is why we end up always being in such pain. Our hip flexors and upper back are tight and extremely weak. Our chest is tight and pulls our shoulders forward. When you have poor posture- you end up with herniated disks, knee problems, ankle problems, and even more. Poor posture leads to all of the above because our bodies actually work together as a whole. Yes, it's true that there are different parts- but all those parts form one whole body.

Following are some of the ways that poor posture can affect your overall health.

## Problems Caused by Poor Posture

You're already aware that your bad posture is causing your shoulders to ache and your neck to creak- but did you realize that it could also be making you grouchy? Following are a few of the strange effects that poor posture has on you overall- along with some tips to help you straighten up.

1. Makes depression worse.

One study at San Francisco State University instructed students to either walk down a hallway skipping or walk down a hallways slouching. Those who were slouching said that they felt an increase in depression and much lower energy levels than those that were skipping. Experts say that even our language reports a connection between emotional affect and posture: a person who is weak is referred to as spineless and someone who is very proud is said to have a backbone.

The way to improve this is to pretend you have a headlight in the middle of your chest. Whether you are sitting or standing, you should make sure your headlight always shines forward. Keep your head over your shoulders and- without lifting your chin, extend your head towards the ceiling

2. Can cause problems with your career.

Slouching not only affects your overall attitude, but can also have an effect on the way people view you. After all, consider this: when you're job searching and going in for interviews, do you really want to go in slouching- or would you rather go in standing tall? Of course you want to go in standing tall because if you go in slouching they're not going to see you as someone they'd want in their company. In order to improve your posture, you want to strengthen the muscles in the middle of your back.

The best way to avoid being a slouch on your job, there is an exercise you can do at your desk: simply lift the bottom of your ribs about an inch or two off of your hipbone. This will pull your shoulder blades down and back. A good way to make sure you maintain this position is to pin a ribbon to the top and the bottom of your shirt and try keeping it taut for about ten minutes at a time- work to increase this each time.

3.  Can cause constipation.

When you are sitting in a crouched/slouched position, your intestines are completely folded up. This slows everything down- which can make you feel bloated/constipated and make you look fat.

Exercises like Pilates and yoga are wonderful for strengthening your core and helping you to keep things moving the way they were meant to. There is one pose that can help you to rev up your sluggish gut: lie down on your belly and rest your head on your lower arms. Then, raise your forehead, looking upwards. This allows your weight to rest on your chest. Allow your head to fall back just a little as you move your belly further up off the ground as if someone is pulling your arms.

4.  Increases your risk of disease and even death.

One recent study in Australia found that after 25 years of age, every hour spent slouching on the couch, watching television reduced an individual's life expectancy by around 21.8 minutes. In addition, when researchers in America cross-referenced this sedate time with health outcomes in another study, those who were more sedate increased their risk of developing conditions such as diabetes and cardiovascular disease- even if they also spent time working out.

You can fix this by not allowing the television to grab you. You can do something called the TV Stand. In this move, you stand up from your chair without pushing yourself up with your hands, and then sit back down in one controlled, smooth motion. This will keep the muscles in your lower body strong.

5. Makes you appear heavier than you really are.

The truth is that we have become a nation that is professional when it comes to sitting. However, when you're slouched, your internal organs go down and out- causing you to look fatter.

You can fix this by simply getting up and moving. When you're standing instead of sitting, you end up burning 20 percent more calories, increase bone density, improve metabolism, and strengthen your muscles.

6. Causes circulation to be cut off.

Be aware that your body is a machine that moves around gases and other fluids. When you sit for a long period of time with your legs crossed, it can cut off this flow, causing spider veins and increased pressure.

In order to get your blood flowing into your lower body, you should stand up and find the best posture for your body. Then, lift one leg so that the thigh is horizontal to the ground. Make sure you keep the leg that you're standing on locked but not hyperextended. Hold for five full, strong breaths, pushing your breaths into your diaphragm.

7. Causes you to be stressed out.

One recent study revealed that those who have a powerful posture- that is straight spines and open shoulders- have an increase in testosterone levels and a decrease in cortisol. However, those who slouch end up decreasing their levels of testosterone and increasing cortisol. This means that you have high stress and low self-confidence. When you sit slouched over your computer, this means shallow chest breathing- which puts stress on your lungs because they must move quicker to ensure that you have proper flow of oxygen- and it puts strain on your heart because it must speed up to provide adequate blood flow to transport the oxygen.

In order to fix this issue, you should remember that those everyday cues such as a stoplight or ringing phone should remind you to combat your stress by taking relaxed abdominal breaths. To check your breathing: place your hand directly below your belly button- your belly should be expanding as you breathe in. invite the air to the deepest portion of your lungs, where the exchange of oxygen is the most efficient. Then, as you breathe out, your belly should contract as stress leaves your body.

Since the body- though it is many parts- works as one system, that is the reason why this program does not focus on thing such as a bicep curl because that is just one isolated movement. Personally, I would rather be moving the entire body, since it works together.

Instead, our focus is primarily on perfecting those movements that we need every single day throughout our lives. This helps us feel better, which ultimately leads to accomplishing more. Therefore- you have better results when you hit the gym.

Secondly, as you saw in "Where Women Go Wrong With Nutrition," our focus has nothing at all to do with calories. Whereas most programs tell you that you must create a caloric deficit in order to lose those pounds, instead we focus on getting the necessary nutrients to properly nourish our bodies. The truth is that people are not really eating too much bad and not enough good- but basically too much food overall.

So, when we look at nutrition, we're not attacking it, saying: "You must stick to this really strict diet." Instead, we choose one thing that can be changed at a time. For example, let's say you're eating Cinnamon Toast Crunch for breakfast, a footlong submarine sandwich for lunch, and fried chicken for dinner- and that's it. You do that every single day of your life.

Our goal is to get you to switch from fried chicken to baked chicken breast with sweet potato and broccoli instead of fried chicken and

French fries one night a week for one month. Then, once you get through the first month, try doing it for two nights a week.

Our approach is a gradual one. We don't jump to those extreme weight loss methods or cleanses. Instead, our focus is on creating habits that help you to properly fuel and nourish your body the way it should be done.

Now, you have a basic understanding of fat loss versus weight loss- which are similar, but very different. You also understand where women tend to go wrong with nutrition and working out- and how our approach to all of this is so much different than the other ones out there.

# The Right Mindset and Goals

In order for a fat loss program to be considered effective, you must have two very simple things:

1. The right mindset

2. Goals

## The Right Mindset

First of all, lets focus on the right mindset. If you are going to work this program, you simply can't come into this thinking, "I'm going to have a six-pack on my abs this time next week."

The truth is, I have been working this program for eight years now. Recently, I posted something online: what I looked like two years ago and where I am now. In the picture from two years ago, you can see that I had let myself go.

When you start this program, you must keep in mind that it's not a quick fix but an establishing of new habits. When you go on those extreme weight loss programs- you must keep in mind two things:

1. You will lose weight- not just fat- meaning that you will lose from your organs, bones, muscles, and more.

2. It will be a yo-yo effect- you'll lose and gain the rest of your life. The cycle will never end.

However, with our program, you're taking your now unhealthy habits and making new, healthy ones. It is going to be part of your everyday life: just like tying your shoes and brushing your teeth. You're not going to have a killer day every single day. Keep in mind that you're going to make mistakes- that's fine. Just don't make those mistakes a reason to quit. Just get right back up, dust yourself off, and start again.

You can maintain this and stay active- but it has to be a regular part of your day. If you start this program, you must keep in mind that this is going to become part of your life. It's not a quick one-, two-, or three-month thing. This will never stop- it will be with you for the rest of your life because it's a habit.

# 3 Mindset Switches

The truth is that each and every person out there has the ability to change their mindsets. Of course, it won't necessarily be a tire-squealing, turn-around switch- but will just be a smooth, drifting change. Here are three mindset switches to get you started:

## 1. *Reverse leadership*

When it comes to losing weight, there is two protocols:

i.   Those who do it privately

ii.  Those who follow-the-leader

The private person secludes themselves and privately tries to go against all those things that keep them from losing weight. the follow-the-leader follows the person that knows more about the subject than they do. There's nothing specifically wrong with either one of these, either of them can work.

However, the problem comes when the follower gets tired of following. This happens in those extreme diets because you're given all kinds of restrictions of what you can and can't do. You're going to get tired of being told you can't have that tiny piece of chocolate- so you end up eating the whole bag.

Instead, there should be a healthy balance of following and leading. You need to take back some of that control from those telling you what to do. That is where our program works. We help guide you in making changes- but you must take control of that and work it for yourself. We're not going to force you to make it happen. The driving force in all of this is YOU!

YOU are the one that can redefine the role you take in losing fat. That is how you will be able to change the way you act and think. This is where your energy- your motivation- will come from.

### 2. Steer your fear.

When it comes to losing weight- fear is a horrible word. We are afraid of the scale. We're afraid of going to the doctor. We're afraid of going shopping. We're afraid of having our pictures taken. However, you should remember that fear causes you to retreat- which makes it that much harder to change our habits and lose that fat that we so desire to rid ourselves of.

The reality is that fear is real- and it's definitely not easy to stop. Still, instead of allowing the fear to steer our actions- we have the ability to steer our fear. There are plenty of writings out there that discuss goal setting and there seems to be a division between setting those BIG goals versus setting those which are more attainable.

The best approach in my opinion is to set at least one mental and physical challenges that is just scary enough to help you make good choices. After all, those good choices will be stepping stones on your path to a healthier, happier, thinner you.

So, what is considered "just enough"? Basically, it is that sweet spot between "YES! I can do this!" and "There's absolutely no way I can do this." The space between those two extremes is where you will grow. Okay, so maybe it's not "fear" in the traditional sense- but the uncertainty is different (and healthier) than the fear that dieters typically have.

### 3. Crank up your voltage.

When it comes to slimming down, having the right mindset is what is going to make you successful. That is the basis of our program. Those small choices and changes you make will- over time- start changing the way you act, look, and feel. No, it's not going to happen overnight.

If you're 60 pounds overweight today- you should not expect to wake up next week 60 pounds slimmer.

However, when it comes to working out- as you already saw- it's not necessarily slow and steady that will get it done. It is whole body, sometimes high-intensity, workouts. We must work as hard as we can because when you're so immersed in your activity, it's fun and intense. It feels good. It feels enjoyable. We're in the moment and it gives us that post-workout endorphin high that keeps us burning calories and helps us to make healthy choices- especially when it comes to food.

Working out, like eating a meal, should never feel like a chore. Instead, in order for it to be effective over time, it must feel more like recess (having fun) than detention (punishment). Allowing yourself to go all in with activity gets you excited enough to get out of your head and want to do it over and over. The byproduct of playing hard is that you reach that goal that you wanted to.

## What are Goals?

A goal is something that you want to work towards. When there is absolutely nothing that you are reaching for, it can be extremely hard to keep your motivation going. For example, when it comes to eating, you should be thinking: "Okay, I'm going to eat healthy, clean meals for one full week- then I'll have a big cheat meal." Then, get through the week and give yourself the reward of that cheat meal.

Or, if your goal is to lose 5 pounds in 30 days, that is something to work towards. However, instead of losing 5 pounds, you should be thinking: "I want to lose 5 pounds of body fat in 30 days."

Once you have reached one goal- set another one and keep it going. You should have long term and short term goals. The short term goals are set for short periods of time that are easily attainable and keep you moving towards your ultimate, long-term goal. This helps you keep your motivation and keep you from giving up.

# Goal Setting

While the primary focus of this book is fat loss- and becoming a healthier you- let's take a moment to review some basic information on goal setting and go over some tips to help you reach those goals.

Let's think about it: have you ever really taken the time to set goals at any point in your life? Think about this: what would you like to achieve in the next year? What about the next three years? Where would you like to be five years from now? What about ten years from now? Are there any aspirations that you're looking forward to coming true?

Taking the time to SET goals for yourself in your fat loss program is the very first step towards successfully achieving those goals. After all, if you have nothing to work towards, then what exactly are you doing, anyway? It is your roadmap that points you in the direction of success. This is the step that will give you the focus and will spur you on to action. Without taking this vital step, you will never achieve anything.

Think about it: have you ever met someone who has a passive approach towards their life? They never set any goals for themselves- they just live life "by the seat of their pants" and whatever happens, just happens. You see them a year from now, even ten years from now, and their lives will basically be exactly the same as they are now, with a few minor changes due to the desires and actions of others more than their own.

Following are six reasons that setting goals for yourself is so vital.

*1. Setting goals gives you clarity.*

If you don't have goals, you're spending life just running and never achieving anything. Of course, you'll have the illusion that you're doing lots of things. However, these things aren't what you'd like to be doing. You're basically just making yourself crazy with making everyone else's goals come true. This could mean that you're working in a career that you don't enjoy simply because you're making money. By doing this, you're making the company's goal come true because they're not having to look for someone else to replace you.

After all, how can you get what you want if you're not setting goals for yourself? How can you reach your visions/dreams if you don't admit the end result you'd like to see. Setting goals for yourself will give you a clear vision of what you ultimately want. Setting goals helps to make you realize the desires you have in your heart and mind. Setting goals will help you to be sure that you're spending your time, talents, and energy in something that really matters. Setting goals makes you live more consciously.

Keep in mind that everything in the world has two creations. The first creation is the mental creation. This is when you THINK about what it is that you wish to achieve. The second creation is the reality. This is when you MAKE IT HAPPEN- when those dreams come true. Without the first creation, there will be no second. Setting a goal takes care of the mental creation. Setting a goal means that you have put into motion the action plan that will help your goal to manifest into reality.

### 2. *Setting goals drives you.*

The goals that you set for yourself are a representation of the desires that give you the drive and the motivation to keep going. The time that you take to set your goals is one of the points in time when you're connected the deepest with the source of your motivation. This is the time that your motivation is at its highest. Having goals are a reminder of your sources of motivations. They are what will keep driving you forward when things get difficult- and they will.

When I feel like I have lost my motivation (and yes, it happens to the best of us), I begin to meditate and direct my focus on the goals that I believe are most important in my life. I take the time to visualize a scenario of my goals being fulfilled- and put so much effort in it that I feel like it's currently happening. Taking the time to do this forms a very clear connection with my desires. Then, my motivation soars, and I am able to use it in my daily actions and life.

### 3.  *Setting goals gives focus.*

Setting goals for yourself will give you something to focus on. A PURPOSE in life gives you a basic direction to focus in. However, GOALS give you something specific to put your focus on. Your time, energy, and effort is the input and the results of your efforts is your output. The goal that you set is the funnel that guides your input to create the output that you desire.

Without goals, you're just moving through life- putting forth a lot of input, but never really achieving any valuable output. You randomly put your energy into activities that you take part in every day. However, these activities are pointless- they don't really man anything in the big scheme of things in your life. You don't realize this, though, because you're just living life as it comes.

Therefore, you end up misconstruing "fun-to-do" activities as "important" activities. You may be taking part in these activities because there's nothing else you can think of to spend your time on.

If you think about it, you may have a general idea of what you'd like to see happen in your life. However, unless you take the time and put forth the effort to define these general ideas into specific goals, you're not going to be funneling your efforts correctly. You'll see that you get sidetracked because you don't have any concrete goals to keep you focused.

It can be really easy to get sidetracked by everyday life. After all, there are so many things out there that can stimulate us. Of course, you may believe that you're moving in the direction of your general desires- but this is an illusion. Without specific goals, you will not have focus. Without the focus, your input will just be random and strewn out- and will not lead to the output you desire.

### 4.  *Setting goals gives you accountability.*

When you have goals in place, there is something there to hold you accountable for your actions. Instead of just talking about what you want and not making the effort to make them come true, you will be required to take action steps. Setting goals will give you a clear idea of whether or not you're actually living for your desires.

Of course, this accountability is only to yourself- not to others. This is what will keep you focused when you choose to drink a glass of water instead of a glass of wine. This is what will keep you focused on your work tasks instead of being distracted by the internet. Keeping yourself accountable with your goals helps you to keep true to your desires.

5.  *Setting goals helps you be the best you that you can be.*

When you set goals, you're setting yourself up to achieve your highest potential. Without having goals, you're just holding yourself back in your comfort zone. This comfort zone, though, will keep you from growing. It will not allow you to become the best you that you can be. It keeps you from reaching that potential that you hold inside.

Setting goals helps you to set up targets that you can strive for. These goals will push you to venture to new places, meet new people, and therefore, place you in situations where there is potential for growth. Goals make you reach past yourself and therefore get to new heights. For example, if you want to lose weight, setting that goal will make your efforts effective. Setting a goal for your career will keep you from settling for something else.

Goals will bring you face-to-face with barriers and push you to get past them. The will make you more aware of yourself and your actions.

6.  *Setting goals helps you live the best life possible.*

When you set goals, you're setting yourself up to get the best out of life. This is due to two reasons:

First of all, setting goals helps you to become a better person. You'll learn more about yourself and your abilities. You will experience more out of the everyday, mundane events of life. Take a moment to consider your personal worldview: how is it different now as compared to ten years ago? Chances are that you see much more clearly now than you did then- I know I do!

Second, no matter how much we try to stop the clock, time keeps ticking away. By setting goals with specific deadlines will help you to be sure that you're maximizing your input and getting your expected output.

As mentioned, you'll need to know your purpose in life in order to come up with your goals. Goals will help you to get the best out of your overall purpose.

Start Setting Your Goals

Now that you understand the reasons for setting goals, it's time to start setting them. Take a moment to ask yourself this: What are my personal goals for the next year? What about three years? What about five years? What about ten?

If you really take the time to set your goals now, you will definitely grow as a person. When you spend just a little bit of time verbalizing some aspirations you've had on your mind, you'll make more progress in your life in one year than you will if you don't do this.

## Tips to Help You Achieve Your Goals

Now that you've learned how you should go about setting your goals, now you need some tips for making those goals come to fruition. After all, there's no point in taking the time and making the effort to set them if you're not going to take some steps to achieve them.

1. Commit yourself to achieving them.

First of all, you must realize that achieving your goals will require lots of dedication and commitment. There's no way to avoid this. If there's a specific goal that you're having trouble committing to, go back to the beginning and start over. It may be that you didn't really identify your goal correctly- or perhaps you're just basically lacking in the motivation to make it happen.

2.   Track your progress to achieving your goals.

You already know that it's important to take the time to write your goals down, right? Now, you must realize that it's just as important to write down your progress to achieving those goals. There are goal tracking worksheets you can get that can help you do this, or apps for your phone/tablet/computer, or any other system that you can come up with. The whole point in tracking your progress is to periodically check on yourself and see where you were, where you need to go, and where you are. This will help you to make sure you're on the right track and you're not completely going off into left field.

3.   Break down the goals you're trying to achieve.

Sure, it's wonderful to have ambitious goals. However, sometimes, those really big, ambitious goals can be quite difficult to achieve. Still, if you take the time to break them down into a group of smaller goals, will make reaching that big goal much more manageable.

4.   Get some help achieving your goals.

Oh, I totally understand, you're independent and want to do it all on your own. Believe me, I tend to be that way myself. However, reaching out to others for support or guidance of some sort in achieving your goals can be a huge help. Perhaps you need someone that can hold you accountable. Even though your goals are very personal to you, the truth is, you're not alone- reach out to someone that you love and trust to help you to achieve those goals. This will make things so much easier.

5.   Be flexible about achieving your goals.

So, you've set your goals and you've made your plan for achieving them. However, perhaps the plan you've made isn't really working that well. The check-in process is the perfect time to revisit and revise your goals and your plan. It's perfectly okay to make some changes, as long as they support the process rather than detract from it.

6. Keep focused on achieving your goals.

Especially when it comes to your long term goals, it's very important that you keep your focus on the big picture. Sure, there will be times when you'll be focused only on what is in front of you and what you're currently doing to achieve your goals. However, it's vital that you keep your destination in mind so that you're not distracted by other things. Plus, when you think about being successful, your motivation is much more likely to stay intact.

7. Be consistent with your actions to achieving your goals.

Two things that are very important when it comes to achieving your goals are consistency and routine. The more routine you make the process, the easier it is to keep it going. You don't want to always be changing the times when you check-in, or any other part of the process.

8. Let your goals grow as you do.

The truth is, things are always changing- your goals will need to change as you do. There may be some short-term goals that you have in mind- but if you make them the "be-all-end-all" you may miss out on something great for your current business, or even personal changes/ changes in society. Make sure that you always keep your goals realistic and relevant- allow them to grow and change as you do.

9. Always be positive on your way to achieving your goals.

Okay, so maybe it sounds a bit cliché, but always thinking on the positive will help to propel you to success. Always thinking negative thoughts will actually ruin the whole process of achieving your goals. However, when you hit a roadblock or a challenge of some sort- and you will- thinking positive thoughts will help you to get past them.

10. Celebrate all of your successes on your way to achieving your goals.

You can't honestly expect your motivation to stay up without rewarding yourself for milestones along the way. Rewarding yourself is a boost to your morale. Not rewarding yourself will bring down your morale and will end up diminishing the entire process of working toward your goals. So, no matter how big or small your progress, make sure to reward yourself along the way.

Of course, when it comes right down to it- while you definitely need the right mindset and the right, attainable goals- your primary focus should be on your personal mindset. After all, your mindset is what is going to keep you determined and focused on meeting those goals. The ones who will achieve positive results are those that stick with it.

In addition, the second focus is not exactly what IS in the book but what is NOT in the book. You'll find that your success is nearly proportionate to keeping the essentials in your program and getting rid of everything else. Basically, you're "trimming the fat" out of your program. The truth is that, in order to lose fat, you don't need any smoke and mirror exercises. You don't need anything fancy. You just need yourself and your commitment to reaching your goals.

# Getting Toned

So far, we've discussed the general idea of fat loss versus weight loss. While the two are often used interchangeably, they are actually two very different concepts. Then, we talked about the mistakes that are made with regards to nutrition and working out- and the best ways to fix both of those. We discussed how our approach to fat loss is different than anything else you might find out there and how you can change your mindset and set attainable goals.

Now, it's time to talk about getting toned. After all, the next step after losing that unnecessary fat is toning your muscles. That is what nearly every one of my clients has asked for after losing fat is help with toning. Information for getting toned is all over the place: internet, books, magazines, and so much more. The toning stage is much different than the fat loss stage.

Toning is where you build up those lean, sexy muscles where that excess fat used to be. When you build up those muscles, there's something that's really nice to look at, right? While it's true that your overall goal may be different- such as the first client listed in "Some Sample Results", the principles are still the same.

You must get yourself back to the basics. I'm sure you've heard the old saying, "the only thing that separates the experts from everyone else is that the experts have mastered the basics."

Once you have taken the time and effort to master the basics, what you will be doing is continuing to challenge yourself. You can challenge yourself by exploring new and different skills, adding different weights to the same movements, or increasing the time that you're able to complete a specific tasks.

One of the most common mistakes is that people simply do not challenge themselves enough. Following are some of the other common mistakes that people make when getting their bodies in shape:

### 1. *They rest too much*

Rest is very important during a workout and is often an overlooked aspect. Resting too long will cause your body to "go cold", essentially undoing your warm up. You have to keep your body warm and ready to go. Resting too little can inhibit performance in upcoming sets. We always go for quality over quantity, so its important to know the proper rest depending on the activity you are doing."

### 2. *They do long, slow workouts*

When you're working out, you need to be focusing on maximizing your time. Certain types of exercise require certain amounts of time. That means that the length of your workout can change depending on what you are doing. After your warm up, start off with your specific strength training. Rest time between these sets should be longer, sometimes 2-4 minutes. When you move on and begin your accessory work, pick up the tempo. Perform complexes with multiple exercises and minimal rest between sets. No more than 1 minute, preferably 30-45 seconds. You want to keep the heart rate up and the blood flowing to your muscles.

### 3. *They improperly lift weights*

If you wish to get toned, you should find a weight that you will be able to lift six to ten times instead of twenty or more. of course, this does not mean to simply stop lifting somewhere between ten and twelve times- it means that the weight you choose should be light enough to where you can do at least ten reps. On the other hand, if you're able to complete more than twelve, the weight is much too light. Once you have found the right weight, you can do one, two, or three sets of each.

### 4. *They don't challenge themselves*

Okay, so you know that when you do the same thing over and over causes you to get bored with it, right? Well, guess what? Your body works the same way. When you get into a routine where you're doing either using the same weights or not learning new things, it becomes much easier and your body gets used to it. This means that the workout is not as effective. This means that the workout is no longer effective. The workout ends up not being challenging anymore and your body ends up using less energy when you do work out. However, when you mix things up and you frequently change your workouts, you actually trick your body into working much harder, building more muscle, and burning more fat.

So, next time you start wondering why you're not seeing results from all the working out you're doing, consider these common mistakes and if you are making one or more of them- then change what you're doing. After all, your body does adapt and you must be able to recognize that you have to keep changing things up to ensure that you keep getting results.

Consider this example: you can squat a 15-pound kettlebell 10 times. It's challenging, but not nearly as challenging as it was when you first started. So now maybe we will either, one, increase how many we do – within reason of course – and when I say to do as many as we can do maybe we won't do 10 times, we'll do 12 or 15 times. Or we'll increase the weight and go for the same number of repetitions that we have been. If you continue to do the same thing at the same intensity for months and months, you won't see the results you're looking for.

As we mentioned earlier, the body adapts incredibly quickly. It needs change and it needs to be challenged. Look for ways to make what you're already doing more difficult and look for ways to challenge yourself by learning new skills and techniques. An example of this could be like the pistol squat, which is being able to squat down on one leg instead of two. So if you're proficient in a lot of other different squat variations, but you don't have the strength or the balance and techniques to perform a full-rep pistol squat, maybe that's what you start to practice. You find a coach who can teach it to you, make sure you're proficient in the regular squat variations, and then you can start practicing the pistol squat. Instead of doing the same thing you always have done for squats, you practice your technique for that one. And that's just one example. There's thousands, millions of other things that you can do with that.

Once we've also gotten through kind of the workout part and we've lost a lot of fat, one thing that really people mess up is their recovery. And their recovery includes everything from water to nutrition to really importantly sleep. If you want to build lean, sexy muscle that kind of pops like those big blocky abs and you want your arms to look nice and your back to look good and your sides to have definition to them, you have got to be eating right and most importantly you've got to be getting good quality sleep and enough of it. That is probably one of the most overlooked aspects of training and fitness is how much sleep people are getting, and it's probably one of the number reasons why people are overweight today. I'm actually pretty convinced that people could start to lose fat just by getting more sleep at night. That's just me.

## Keys to Getting Toned

There are five keys to getting toned:

1.  **Recovery: you must allow your body to recover properly. This entails getting adequate rest.**

So number one: recovery and sleep. Some people sleep better than others. I have some off-sleep patterns, and sometimes I sleep great. You should try and find a way that you are ... kind of like a little ritual in the p.m. that kind of gets you set up to sleep. It's not really good to just get home from work and go right to bed. That's hard to do. But you really do need to get enough sleep. I say six hours is an absolute minimum for me. I will put off everything else – I'll put off work and whatever, I'll put off my workout – if I'm not able to get six hours of sleep. So you want to be aiming for at least seven to eight hours of sleep to make sure you are recovering as well as you can. And I mean, like eight hours of shut-eye, not two hours of fiddling around on an iPad and then six hours of, okay, I'm asleep now. In the next chapter, we'll talk about the things that could be causing you to not sleep and how you can change those habits/problems.

2.  **Eating Right: when you choose your meals, you should be eating the right foods and eating as little as you possibly can of those foods that are not good for you.**

Number Two: Eating enough of the right foods and as little as possible of the bad foods. So are you eating colorful vegetables? I say colorful vegetables because French fries are not a vegetable. You want your broccoli, your asparagus, your carrots, your cauliflower, your spinach, your kale – all that kind of stuff. Are you eating enough of that along with lean proteins to help fuel the body? That's what the body needs to nourish itself. And are you eating as little as possible of the bad foods? Cake, candy, soda, alcohol, ice cream, sugar in general. What are you drinking in your coffee? It blows my mind that people are so quick to denounce eggs because they're *so terrible for you*, but they'll go to Starbucks and get some loaded up caramel macchiato with all this sugar in it. I don't think your eggs are the problem. I'm pretty sure we could fix your coffee and you'd see significant results! So things like that, where are you getting things that you don't need? Where are you getting all this sugar that maybe you are conscious about and maybe you're not conscious about? Maybe you didn't know that your coffee is bad for you and you should really just be having plain black coffee with a little bit of milk in it. That's not bad for you at all – that's actually pretty good for you.

3.  **Build strength & challenge yourself: you should be taking the time to build up your strength and looking for new ways to challenge yourself.**

Number three is: getting strong – so you want to be able to, one, control your own body weight, and then two, get proficient in the basic human movements, which are hinge, squat, push, pull and carry. So, you want to be able to pick something off the ground. That's a hinge. You want to be able to stand up with something on your back – that's just general sitting down and standing up each day. Pushing and pulling is pretty self-explanatory. You need to be able to push yourself off the ground with your hands – let's say you fall – or to pull yourself up if you're hanging up from something and you need to pull yourself back up to a stable base. And then carrying, the most basic thing that anybody ever does, carrying your groceries from the car into the house. Carrying your kids around. What if you have to move? You need to be able to carry some of your things to one house to the other and help the movers, things like that. Constantly challenge yourself. So don't settle.

When I can squat 20 pounds, all right, let's go to the next one. Let's squat 25 pounds. You can't just settle for a weight and a lot of people tend to do that, because they see the number and they're like, "Oh, no, that's too much for me." We have plenty of people that are lifting well over weight they ever thought they'd lift for.

4. **New skills: take the time and make the effort to learn some new skills so that you don't get bored with your workout or it becomes ineffective.**

Number Four: learn new skills, like I mentioned before, the pistol squat. I'll give an example of one of my close friends, who she is in her early 30s and she's in really good shape. She's been working out with me for a long time. She was never really overweight or had a lot of fat to lose. She wanted to get stronger and she wanted to get better. So we got her better and we got her feeling good and she was like, "I want to start to do some things that I can't do right now." And I was like, "Well, what's something that you can't do that you've always wanted to do?" And she said her sister was a gymnast and she wasn't. And her sister used to walk around on her hands and things like that. So we were like, "All right, let's get you good at handstands. Let's start doing stuff like that." Now, she's an experienced person in the gym, so we can work with her at that level. That's not something that we do with a brand new person or somebody even one or two years into it. She's five to six years into working out with me and has always been in fairly good shape. That's just a skill that she's never been able to do before, so she's working on it.

Over the years of my extensive study and training, I have learned that kettlebells seem to work best- especially for women. As the fitness industry begins to grow more and more, kettlebells are gaining popularity.

The thing that is so wonderful about kettlebells is that all the movements that kettlebells are used for are those basic movements that we just talked about, those basic human movements. The kettlebell helps make these movements incredibly inefficient, and what I mean by that is they pretty much waste energy, and they're perfect for really ... wasting energy is the way to burn fat. Burning that fat for energy while combining that with a strength movement. So you can actually get stronger and lose fat doing kettlebells at the same exact time. And that's really what you want- and it keeps it lean.

So a lot of women are really concerned about bulking and they don't want to lift weights because they're going to get too bulky – which is never going to happen – and what kettlebells do is it really helps keep that muscle lean and not get too big as far as what they would like to see.

# Sleep to Lose Fat

That's right- you definitely read that right. One of the reasons why you may not be losing fat is because you're not getting the sleep that you need. When you don't get enough sleep, you are causing your metabolism to slow down- which keeps you from burning that excess fat. Your body is holding on to it because it needs that extra fuel to keep going during the day.

## Why Aren't You Sleeping?

If you don't get a good night's sleep, you are more than likely going to have a very difficult time waking up and getting motivated to own your day. So, let me extend this wakeup call to you- if giving up a good night's sleep is the first thing you're giving up, you're not just making it difficult for you to function the next day. Ultimately, you're actually doing some serious damage to your overall health.

Sleep deprivation is actually a very serious medical risk that very few people are actually aware of. However, the truth is, you must pay just as much attention to your sleep patterns as you do to your diet and exercise.

Studies are revealing that there are some pretty clear links between not getting enough sleep and being overweight or even obese. In addition, there have been studies that have shown that there is a correlation between sleep deprivation and heart disease, type 2 diabetes, and hypertension. On the other hand, experts are saying that if you can start getting enough sleep, you can reverse these conditions.

When we take the time to figure out what exactly robs us of restful sleep, experts have come up with some strategies that can help you get the rest that is necessary to keep your body going and help you to wake up and get motivated in the mornings. This chapter will provide you with some of the things that are keeping you from being able to get good sleep and how you can ban them from the bedroom so that you will be able to dominate your day and sleep through your nights.

### 1. *You're thinking entirely too much.*

One of the major reasons you're obsessing over that problem at work or perhaps an argument with your best friend or your spouse when you're falling asleep is that you're not able to redirect your thoughts when you're falling asleep like you can when you're wide awake. Since you're drifting in and out of sleep, though you think you're fully awake, you're not able to have the control that you need over your thoughts to keep yourself from worrying.

Tips to Fix this Problem

If you're having trouble falling asleep because of worries, get up and leave your bedroom. However, don't turn on any lights. Chances are, when you're up and moving, these worries will dissipate and you'll be able to go right back to bed and fall asleep. This strategy is known as stimulus control and it also helps to keep you from associating your bed with worry.

Another strategy is to set aside a time in the evening- before going to bed- to work on some problem solving. Get a notebook and a pen and jot down the worries that are weighing you down as well as one to two possible solutions for each one. You should do this a few hours before going to bed.

### 2. *You're sleeping in.*

As mentioned in the previous chapter, spending your weekends staying up or out late and sleeping in the next morning will definitely wreak havoc on your internal clock. This internal clock is controlled by a nerve cell cluster in your bran that also controls your body temperature and your appetite. Then, by the time Sunday comes, you've already reprogrammed your body to stay up well past your normal bedtime and then on Monday, you have difficulty waking up in the morning and getting motivated- so you can't dominate your day.

Tips to Fix this Problem

Even if you stay out late with friends on Friday or Saturday night, get up at your normal time the next morning. If you must sleep in a little later, don't sleep more than one hour past your normal wake up time. In order to catch up on the sleep you lost by staying up, you can take a short catnap in the afternoon- but don't sleep for more than thirty minutes because that can keep you from falling asleep that night.

*3.   Your spouse snores.*

Did you know that a snorer can reach around 90 decibels, which is as loud as a blender? So, even if you are able to fall asleep, this snoring will likely wax and wane all through the night, causing you to wake up during the most restful phase of sleep, REM.

Tips to Fix this Problem

Talk to your spouse about his or her snoring and ask if it's possible for them to sleep on their back. You can even purchase a special pillow that was created by a neurologist from Harvard. This pillow is shaped specially to tilt your head and to open up your airways and has proven to decrease- and even eliminate snoring in almost all patients studied and also reduced the occurrence of sleep interruptions from 17 or more to 5 or less.

On the other hand, if this doesn't work, you can always use earplugs. These can be very effective, as long as they stay in.

*4.   Changes in your hormones.*

The levels of progesterone and estrogen in women tend to fluctuate either before or during your period and even during perimenopause and can cause sleep problems. Chances are, you're going to notice that you're having difficulty sleeping- typically waking up through the night- a long time before you start experiencing hot flashes.

Tips to Fix this Problem

If you often are awakened by cramps during your period, take an OTC pain reliever when you go to bed or take a hot bath a couple of hours before going to bed. Chances are, this may be all that you need to deal with that premenstrual insomnia.

If the above treatments don't help, you can speak with your physician to see if he or she would recommend a short acting sleep medication for you to take two to three times a month.

When you're going through perimenopause, try to make sure that you stay on a consistent schedule, get at least twenty to thirty minutes of exercise per day, and stay away from caffeine or alcohol at least three hours before going to bed. Sure, the alcohol will help you to fall asleep, but it will cause you to wake up later in the night.

If you're suffering from night sweats and hot flashes, try to keep your room as cool as possible and wear light pajamas. If this doesn't work, consider speaking with your physician about hormone therapy. Some research has shown that hormone therapy could actually be safe for women in their 50s, especially when they use it for less than five years.

### 5. You're hungry.

If you go to bed hungry, that will definitely interfere with your ability to get quality, restorative sleep. Hunger pangs will definitely wake you up. Some studies have revealed that individuals who are dieting will have frequent episodes of waking throughout the night.

Tips to Fix this Problem

When you're dieting, you should reserve some of your calories for a protein packed bedtime snack such as a hard-boiled egg or even a small glass of 2% milk. Proteins will keep you full and allow you to sleep, whereas a snack of fat or carbohydrates will not.

### 6. You have a messy bedroom.

If your bedroom is a cluttered mess, that makes for a cluttered mind. When your mind is cluttered, it is likely to churn throughout the night because you're so stressed. The number one cause of short term insomnia or waking throughout the night is stress.

#### Tips to Fix this Problem

The best way to clear the clutter is to grab a basket and toss in any unfinished work such as bills, that unfinished scrapbook, or spreadsheets and put it away. After all, out of sight, out of mind. If you can't see it, you're less likely to worry about it.

Also, it's best if you have your computer in another room- but if this isn't possible, keep it in a cabinet that can be closed. This will help you to effectively close the door on stress and late-night screen gazing, which studies have proven really does hinder sleep. The bright display of your computer monitor will keep your body from naturally producing melatonin, which is the hormone that is responsible for letting your body know that it is time to go to bed.

### 7. Your room is glowing.

Something you may not realize is that the ambient light from your DVD player, alarm clock, or even the streetlight outside your bedroom window could be responsible for keeping you awake. Even a very small amount of light can enter your retina even when your eyes are closed. This small amount of light can disturb your internal clock and cause you to wake up.

#### Tips to Fix this Problem

If there is a light in the hallway outside your bedroom, close the door. You can also turn your alarm clock to face the wall or get an analog clock (or you can just cover it up like I do). Finally, don't have a night light. You can also purchase one of those old-fashioned eye masks to tell your brain that it is time to sleep.

If the light is coming from outside, you can purchase blackout curtains and shades which can either be attached to your current window treatments or hung up on their own.

### 8. It's too quiet.

Some people will tell you that any sound at all- traffic, rowdy neighbors, or the television- will keep them from sleeping soundly at night. On the other hand, there are others who say that lack of sound keeps them from sleeping- typically, these are those individuals who live in the city.

Tips to Fix this Problem

Believe it or not, it's not that the lack of sound or the sound itself is keeping you from getting quality, restorative sleep. The thing that is disruptive to your sleep cycle is the fact that the sound is inconsistent.

You can turn on an exhaust fan or a ceiling fan to create a white noise, which will block out those disruptive noises and will also provide just enough noise for those that can't sleep in total silence. You can also purchase a white noise machine- or download an app on your phone- to help you get the sleep that your body craves so that you can wake up early the next morning.

### 9. You have dust mites in bed with you.

Whether you realize it or not, chances are that you are sharing your bed with somewhere between 100,000 to ten million dust mites. The residue left behind by these dust mites can cause you to experience mild to severe allergies.

Tips to Fix this Problem

If you want to reduce your allergies, you should make sure that you're dusting and vacuuming on a regular basis. Consider purchasing and using linens that block dust mites, and if your mattress is older than ten years old, you should replace it.

Also, you can crack your doors and windows, which increases the airflow in the room and therefore reduces the occurrence of dust mites.

### 10. You let your pet sleep with you.

Sure, you love your pet- and over half of animal owners admitted that they allow their pet to sleep with them, which results in a disruption of sleep.

### Tips to Fix this Problem

Instead of allowing your dog sleep in the bed with you, get a crate and place it beside your bed, letting him or her sleep there. The American Kennel Club states that dogs enjoy sleeping in a safe and protected area.

On the other hand, if you have a cat, lock him or her out with special toys for the nighttime and put those away in the morning. To keep your cat from scratching at the door, put double sided tape on the bottom edge- cats can't stand the sticky feeling.

As you see, there are lots of things that can keep you from getting the restorative rest that you need. If you're not getting adequate sleep, you're going to have trouble waking up in the mornings. If you can't wake up and get motivated, chances are that you're not going to dominate your day- but your day will dominate you.

# Getting Started with Our Program

The big secret to losing fat and getting in shape is to take things one step at a time. When we are getting someone started on our program, we take the time to assess where they are before they do anything at all. After all, someone that is brand new to fitness is not going to be able to jump into a program as readily as someone who has been training for years.

We use a scale- and I don't mean a weight scale- that tells you if you're not working out at all right now- you should get started with one day per week. Once you have mastered working out once a week, move to two days. Move along at that pace until you are working out every day of the week.

In addition to figuring out where you are on the continuum, you must find a much deeper sense of the reasoning why you want to lose fat and get in shape. After all, if you go into this simply wanting six-pack abs, it's not likely to work out because that's a superficial reason.

On the other hand, a deeper reason would be to stay healthy for your children- this would be a much more powerful motivator. Since there are lots of moms in our program, that's typically what most of them use as their motivation. They want to stay healthy for their kids. They want to be able to run around with their kids and play with their kids- and even their grandkids. So, that's what really makes it, I guess, enjoyable, because they feel like they're doing something worthwhile.

Also, I just try to keep the atmosphere fun and light and once people sort of get into it, most people – I would say nine out of 10 people – enjoy seeing themselves do things and accomplishing tasks that they never thought that they could before. So I think that helps out a lot, and then of course I just try to be entertaining as well.

So most of the people that step into my gym have no idea what they are doing. Even if they think they know. They've worked out before but they aren't seeing results. Why? Because they aren't doing the right exercises with the right load in the right amount of time with the correct form. I always compare it to the doctor. How often are you able to self-diagnose any kind of sickness, aside from the common cold, and give yourself the proper treatment? You would probably get better a lot quicker letting the doctor examine you and prescribe you the correct medication.

That's what DEA Strength is. We're the fat loss doctor and we're here to help you feel and look better, sooner rather than later. So I ask people to look at me like, "Listen, your problem is you don't like the way you look, you don't like the way you feel. I'm going to examine where your problems are in that area and I'm going to give you a prescription.

Now you're going to be able to come here and you're going to be able to know exactly what to do, when to do it, how much to use, and you're going to do it with the right form," instead of going into any other gym and not knowing what's going on, thinking, "Hey, I'm getting into the gym. Walking through the door must magically give me results." So that's what we do differently than others.

## About Our Atmosphere

In our program, the atmosphere is really all about the people. They are our everything. Of course it all starts with the trainer, but having people there that you essentially, they're not just clients. They're friends and they get to know everybody else and we really try to facilitate a close community and getting to know one another.

When you become friends with those that you're working out with, they hold you accountable and make you look forward to working out because they are there to give you the encouragement you need, help you learn, and you're all working together for a common end goal.

Also, sometimes, some people like a little competition, so every now and then we'll get some competition between friends going on, and that's always fun too. But it's really about the people in there and you've got to make sure that that atmosphere with those people is facilitated correctly. So of course having the right kinds of music on, the trainer having energy, making sure that people get to know one another, and that's just through general conversation. Every single day I will ask everybody what was the best and worst part of your day? And sometimes it gets kind of interesting, but people kind of get to know each other through that. And it's a lot of fun. And that really is what brings in the people wanting to get … it's so much better than having to go walk around a treadmill with your headphones in your ears by yourself for an hour.

## The Power of Community

In our program, as you can see, we are about creating a sense of community. After all, the power of community is everything. We would be nothing, really, without our community. Community gives everyone a sense of worth and value, and this is, I mean, that just means so much. It becomes more than just another check on your to-do list for the day, and that's what we want.

People want to come to the gym because they feel important and wanted there and like they belong to something. All of us want something like that. It's really; it makes us look like we're something that people desire to be a part of, and that we're doing more than just selling training. Like we care about each other, we're here to help each other. Because when we're all better, we can all help more people.

## Why Do People Return?

The reason people keep coming back to our gym and our program is because they are seeing results. They are feeling better and looking better. They also come back because they enjoy the sense of community we create and it gives them an escape from their everyday life.

# The Winner's Mindset

As we mentioned earlier in the book, having the right mindset is crucial to your success in our program. If you don't have the right mindset, nothing else that you've read so far really matters, right? So, how can you get a winner's mindset?

The winner's mindset is pretty plain and simple. It is a combination of two ideas:

1. Slow and steady wins the race

2. You can accomplish anything

Basically, a winner's mindset keeps you gong- no matter what- even if you have setbacks. You simply have to take it one step at a time, do one rep at a time, put one foot in front of the other. Then, you must believe in yourself- have confidence that while you might not be able to do a particular move right now, eventually you will be able to do it- but you have to keep trying. You must keep trying until you are able to succeed.

In my experience, if you don't believe that you can do something, chances are that you're not even going to put forth the effort. When it comes to health and fitness, you are going to have ups and downs. You are going to have major setbacks and major successes. That's just the way life in general goes.

The important thing is this: no matter what your results are- you must keep going in the direction that you want to. If there is something you're doing that's simply not working, then you must try something else. The key is this: no matter what, never give up. Never walk away from your goals.

The whole idea behind slow and steady is that taking one step at a time, and not giving up at the first sign of a struggle. Which goes hand in hand with believing you can do anything. If you believe it, you can do it. When you believe in yourself, you can accomplish anything because you're willing to try new things- even those things that scare you or that you've never done before. This can be trying heavier weights, jumping on a high box, or even competing in an obstacle course.

One of my favorite quotes is: "Whether you think that you can or you think that you can't, you're probably right." This is the truth. You can- and will- do anything at all that you set your mind to because it's all about your mindset!

There's another quote that I love that was said by Theodore Roosevelt: "And who, at the worst- if he fails- at least fails while daring greatly, so that his place shall never be with those cold and timid souls who neither know victory nor defeat." To me, this means it's better to try and fail that to never try at all- at least you will have done something. After all, it really doesn't matter if you remain complacent and you never try. However, if you try and don't succeed at least you can say that you did SOMETHING.

Nothing will change if you never attempt to make a change. Isn't the definition of insanity doing the same thing over and over and expecting different results? You're not going to lose fat and get in shape if you keep sitting at home day after day watching television and eating popcorn.

You can't let fear of failure keep you frozen. Sure, what if you try something and you fail? So what? What if you don't? What if you are successful and you are able to keep your momentum going? What if that one step leads to a major life change? What then?

## Cultivating a Winner's Mindset

In order to cultivate a winner's mindset, we help our members to create a habit. As we said earlier, this is not a fitness or weight loss program that will get you to your desired results and you just lay it aside. This is a life change- this is a habit- a new way of living.

In order to build on these habits, we have motivators. After all, you need motivation if you intend to keep going, right? High on the list of motivators are children and family. Parents want to be around for their children. Husbands and wives want to be there for each other. So when something extra challenging comes up, I ask a client: "Do you know who you are doing this for? Sure, you're struggling with this and it's tough- but keep in mind who you are doing this for." When I bring up the names of these motivators, it helps to turn on and light the fuse with a "can-do" positive attitude instead of them giving up.

In addition to encouraging them with their motivators, we also encourage our clients to sign up for events. For example, we occasionally do obstacle courses. When they sign up for events, it gets them locked into something, which also motivates them: "I have to do this so I can be ready for that race/obstacle course/etc." This gives them something else to think about besides simply fat loss. They're not simply looking at the number on the scale and they're not just looking in the mirror. They're working towards a goal- which is a much easier way to stay on the path because they're not working out for the sake of working out.

Believe it or not, this winner's mindset translates into the rest of our clients lives as well. They come to me and tell me that they are surprised because they really didn't believe that a workout regimen would actually make them feel so good mentally and emotionally. They tell me that they've never felt so good, never felt so accomplished or confident and that this training has become the best part of their day. This attitude gives them an overall much more positive outlook on the rest of their lives as well because they're actually active now.

After all, this "can-do" attitude is not something they pick up when they enter the gym and put down when they leave. They carry it with them. They start looking for new challenges and ways that they can improve themselves. They are much happier and they finally understand that they are truly in charge of the way they are thinking. After all, if you truly want to be happy, you can be happy. However, you have to take the time and make the effort to cut out all those negative thoughts and thought processes and bring in the positive, happy thoughts.

You must start by telling yourself (even if you don't believe it just yet) OUT LOUD: "I can do this and I am a truly happy person." If you keep repeating this over and over, eventually you will start to believe it and you will come to the realization that it really is true. It is huge for anyone to be able to walk away with this kind of feeling when they've never had it before and is one of the reasons why they choose to keep coming to our gym and our program over and over.

# Some Sample Results

In this book, you have learned the following:

How fat loss and weight loss are different

Mistakes women make regarding working out and nutrition

How this approach is different

Now, it's time to take a look at some of the results that we've seen. Since this program is not an extreme but focuses on taking one step at a time it is quite effective. There are individuals out there who have used this program and have seen some amazing results.

Of course, you should keep in mind that individual results may vary- because everyone is different. Plus, some individuals will put in more work and others will put in less depending upon how committed they are to the program and what other obligations they have in their lives. So, the truth is that you'll get out of it just what you put into it. You'll have to put in the right stuff to get out what you want.

There are two people that stand out in my mind that have achieved results they never thought possible.

### Case Study #1

One of my clients has been with me for around three years. Initially, he lost more than sixty pounds. He was around 235 pounds when he started and now, he is fluctuating between 175 and 180. Sometimes, he even gets down to around 170.

When he first came to us, his body fat was 24 to 25 percent. Now, after working our program, he's around 12 percent. Guess what? This guy just turned 60 years old!

Many times, individuals come to me and say, "I'm too old. I simply can't burn fat as quickly as younger people can." However, this really isn't true at all. Sure, it's going to take more work- but he was dedicated to his goals- and you can be too.

He put his focus on eating the right things, getting stronger, being less sedate, and feeling better overall. In fact, he says that he's feeling so much better now- at the age of 60- than he ever did when he was 25 to 30. This is amazing! He goes around talking about our program and how he is now part of the elite group of athletes that we also work with. He's even able to do some of the same things they do. He's lifting weights that even college kids can't lift.

Again, this guy is 60 years old! I'm not harping on his age- but people are always telling him how great he looks. Now that he's gotten rid of the extra weight, he's focusing more on getting the body he wants- so we're being a little stricter with his diet and fine-tuning some of the other things to help him improve some of the areas that he really wants to. He's been with us for THREE years. This is not something that is going to happen overnight. He has been committed to us and has put forth effort.

### Case Study #2

I have another client that has actually only been with me for around 6 or 7 months. She's only coming twice a week. Sure, that's not a lot, but when she does come in- she hits it hard. She's always up for a new challenge. She's always asking what she can be doing to get more and she's willing to put in the work.

She had a good bit of weight to lose. In fact, she's one of those that her weight could have had devastating effects in a few years. She's in her 30s or 40s and is a mother.

In the few short months she's been working the program, she's lost more than forty pounds. That's just working the program twice a week! She's always on the go- active in many ways.

She's lost a good bit of weight. Her goal was to get below 230 pounds by December and she's definitely surpassed that at this point.

This proves my statement that you're going to get out of it what you put into it. People are now coming on board with our program and pushing their bodies to see what they are capable of- but those are the two that stand out in my mind.

# Conclusion

Thank you again for purchasing this book! I hope that you have learned some valuable information about fat loss versus weight loss. Though we do typically use the terms interchangeably, they are truly two entirely different concepts. When we lose fat, we're trimming inches off our bodies. However, when we lose weight, we're losing it from all over: fat, muscles, bones, and organs.

In order to make this program work, you must adjust your mindset and set your goals. You need an ultimate, long-term goal and several short term goals/steps that you need to achieve to get to that long-term end goal.

We hope that you will make the commitment to change your life for the better. Keep in mind that this is not a "weight loss program" exactly- but an overall, life-changing program. This is not something that you'll do until you lose the fat that you want and then go back to your unhealthy way of life. This is a commitment you'll make for the rest of your life.

I want to leave you with one final thought: you must do something- even if it's just one simple thing. You don't have to go big to get started- small, simple changes will get you going and give you the momentum you need to keep going.

The very first step in the process is to set your long term, ultimate goals. Then, break those down into smaller goals and finally, even smaller steps. When you look at your long term, ultimate goal it can be quite overwhelming. However, you are in control and you will master your goals- one at a time.

Decide what it is that you want and make the commitment to give it all you've got and then you must find someone and something that will help you do just that. Find someone that will be able to keep you accountable. Find your motivation- something and someone that will help keep you moving towards your goals, even when you have setbacks because when you do just ONE thing each and every day towards your overall health and fitness, you will be successful.

The next step is to get started on your fat loss journey. You really can do this!

Thank you and good luck!

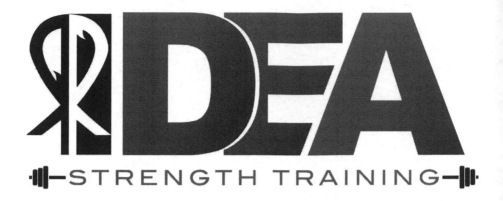

# Free Gift Just For You!

With your purchase of Strength! you get
one week of unlimited access to DEA Strength Training's
Metabolic Conditioning class FREE! (**$50 Value**).

Simply give us a call at 215-400-0866
to reserve your spot today.

Made in the USA
Middletown, DE
25 February 2016